How to Make Bath Bombs

Written by Erin Jones

This book contains material protected under International and Federal Copyright Laws and Treaties. Any unauthorized reprint or use of this material is prohibited. No part of this book may be reproduced or transmitted in any form or by any means, electronic or mechanical, including photocopying, recording, or by any information storage and retrieval system without express written permission from the author.

© 2014 All rights reserved.

Disclaimer:

The information contained in this book is for general information purposes only.

While we endeavor to keep the information up to date and correct, we make no representations or warranties of any kind, express or implied, about the completeness, accuracy, reliability, suitability or availability with respect to the book or the information, products, services, or related graphics contained in the book for any purpose. Any reliance you place on such information is therefore strictly at your own risk.

None of the information in this this book is meant to be construed as medical advice. Essential oils are powerful compounds. Consult with a medical professional prior to making changes that could impact your health.

Contents

Introduction to Bath Bombs   7
Making Your First Bath Bomb   9
Step 1: Mix the Baking Soda and Citric Acid   11
Step 2: Adding the Rest of the Dry Ingredients   14
Step 3: Combine the Wet Ingredients   17
    Carrier Oils   19
    Butters   22
    Essential Oils   24
    Dyes   26
Step 4: Combine the Wet and the Dry Ingredients   27
Step 5: Achieving the Right Consistency   28
Step 6: Molding   30
Step 7: Let the Bath Bombs Dry   32
Step 8: Storage   33
Step 9: Using a Bath Bomb   34
Do Not Use: Sodium Lauryl Sulfate (SLS)   35
Practice Makes Perfect: The Basic Bath Bomb Recipe   36
    Basic Bath Bomb Recipe   36
Oatmeal Bombs   38
    Oatmeal Bombs Recipe   38
Glitter Bombs   40
    Glitter Bombs Recipe   40

Rainbow Sherbet Bath Bombs	42
Rainbow Sherbet Bath Bombs Recipe	42
Lovely Lavender	44
Lovely Lavender Recipe	44
Tea Tree Oil Bath Bomb	46
Tea Tree Oil Bath Bomb Recipe	46
Candy Cane Bath Bombs	48
Candy Cane Bath Bomb Recipe	48
Pink Grapefruit Bath Bombs	50
Pink Grapefruit Bath Bomb Recipe	50
Pear Bath Bombs	52
Pear Bath Bombs Recipe	52
Rose Petal Surprise	54
Rose Petal Surprise Recipe	54
Taste of the Tropics Bath Bomb	56
Taste of the Tropics Recipe	56
Summer Breeze	58
Summer Breeze Bath Bomb Recipe	58
Hot Chocolate Bomb	60
Hot Chocolate Bomb Recipe	60
Skin Softening Bath Bomb	62
Skin Softening Bath Bomb Recipe	62
Skin Toning Bath Bomb	64
Skin Toning Bath Bomb Recipe	64

The Awakening	66
The Awakening Recipe	66
The Goodnight Bomb	68
The Goodnight Bomb Recipe	68

Introduction to Bath Bombs

Every person I know who has tried bath bombs has fallen head-over-heels in love with them. They're one of those items you can go an entire lifetime without knowing they exist, but once you try them they become so ingrained in your daily life that you begin to wonder how you ever lived without them. My friend Jenny compares bathing in a tub with a bath bomb in it to being inside a big bottle of champagne. I prefer to think of it as my own personal mini hot tub with tiny bubbles, except it smells much better and I don't have to worry about catching that rash Aunt Karen has on her elbows.

I'm thinking that if you bought this book you probably already have at least a passing knowledge of what bath bombs are and what they do, but just in case you happened to stumble across this book at a friend's house, here's a quick description.

Bath bombs are little slices of heaven, sent down by the angels above. They're shed from the tips of the angel's wings and float down to Earth at midnight on the third Sunday of Solstice and you have to catch them before they hit the ground or they melt into the Earth never to be seen again. OK, maybe they aren't that special, but when you're sitting in your tub surrounded by bubbles with the smell of essential oils and butters dancing around your nose, tell me it doesn't feel divine.

People tend to think bath bombs are hard to make because they look like they're hard to make. They're formed into interesting shapes and they contain a number of mysterious ingredients like citric acid and essential oils.

They fizz when dropped in the tub, so it's assumed that the fizzing is due to a complex chemical reaction. In reality, bath bombs are surprisingly simple. There are two ingredients in bath bombs that make them fizz and several other ingredients that are added to hold them together, make them smell good and to add therapeutic benefits. All you have to do is combine the ingredients in a certain way, press them into a mold and give them time to dry. A day or two later, you're rewarded with a bath bomb that can be used immediately or stored for later use. Of course it's a little more complicated than that, or this would be the shortest book ever written, but that's the gist of it.

This book was written with the beginner in mind, but contains a lot of good information and is a solid refresher course for the experienced bath bomb maker. It also contains a bunch of recipes that are easy to make and will please beginners and veterans alike.

Making Your First Bath Bomb

We're going to start this book off differently than most guides. Instead of boring you to death with details, we're going to start things off by making a bath bomb to show you how easy it is. You're going to need some supplies, so get a pen and paper and get ready so you can create a shopping list.

You're going to want to gather the following supplies:

- **Baking soda.**
- **Citric acid.**
- **Corn starch.**
- **Salts.**
- **Witch hazel.**
- **Some sort of vegetable oil. Extra-virgin olive oil will work for now.**

That's all the ingredients you're going to need. If you're anything like me, you already have most of these ingredients in your house. The rest can purchased at your local supermarket, drug store, health food store or pharmacy. If you can't find them locally, they can be ordered online.

You're also going to want some essential oils for adding fragrance to the bath bombs. We'll cover the various types of oils you can use in a later chapter, but for now let's go with lavender essential oil. If you don't like lavender, you can use a different essential oil, but it's important to make sure it's safe for contact with your skin. After all, you don't want to dive headfirst into a tub containing essential oil only to find out you're allergic to it. You'll be in for a world of hurt!

While the steps may vary a bit from bath bomb to bath bomb, you're going to be doing pretty much the same thing for every bath bomb you make. Once you've made a few batches and have the process dialed in, it doesn't change much. Making this recipe a couple times before moving on to harder stuff will help you get things dialed in.

Step 1: Mix the Baking Soda and Citric Acid

Baking soda and citric acid are the ingredients that make the magic happen. When you combine them when they're dry, nothing happens. Add moisture to the mix and you get a reaction that creates carbon dioxide. This reaction is what creates the bubbles you see jumping out of the bath bomb when you toss it in the tub. It's kind of like throwing a Gremlin in a swimming pool, only much more relaxing. The bubbling that occurs when a bath bomb comes in contact with water is similar to the carbonation in soda, except bath bombs create much more bubbling action.

Baking soda, aka sodium bicarbonate, aka who cares what the scientific name is, is a naturally-occurring compound that's a white, crystalline solid when found in nature. Since most people wouldn't know what to do with a large chunk of crystal, manufacturers are kind enough to break it up and sell it in powdered form. You probably already have some in your pantry or in a cabinet somewhere. If not, you can buy it at pretty much any store that sells baking supplies. Just don't use that box you've left open in your fridge for the last month to suck up bad smells. You don't want your bath bombs to smell like garlic and old chili. Trust me on this one.

Citric acid is a little bit harder to find. Like baking soda, it's also used in recipes, but it isn't as ubiquitous of an ingredient. It's a weak organic acid found in citrus fruits that's commonly used to preserve cosmetic products. In bath bombs, its sole purpose is to react with the baking soda and to produce bubbles when water is added. It can be found in some supermarkets and may also be available at health food stores and stores that sell supplies to home brewers of beer.

If you don't have access to citric acid, cream of tartar can be used in its place, but you won't get the same bubbling action you do with citric acid. Cut the amount of tartaric acid you use in half when swapping it for citric acid in your recipes.

There's one key rule you need to remember when mixing citric acid and baking soda in Step 1. That rule is you always need to maintain a 2-to-1 ratio of baking soda to citric acid. What this means is if you're making a really tiny bath bomb, you might use 2 tablespoons of baking soda and 1 tablespoon of citric acid. Since I'm sure nobody actually does that, you can also mix 2 cups of baking soda with 1 cup of citric acid. If you're working on a large project, you might mix 2 pounds of baking soda with 1 pound of citric acid. As long as you keep the ratio at 2:1, you're good to go.

When mixing smaller amounts of baking soda and citric acid, it's probably easiest to just dump the two ingredients in a bowl and stir them together until they're thoroughly mixed. When mixing larger amounts, I used to add them to a sifter and sift them into a bowl until one day my husband suggested combining them in one of the shaker jars I use to mix protein drinks in when I actually find time to work out. It worked wonderfully and the shaker jar is my go-to baking soda/citric acid mixer now.

Regardless of the method you use, you're going to want to get rid of all the lumps. Each lump is an area where nothing is mixed together, and if you leave the lumps in the mixture, the bath bombs won't fizz the way you expect them to. If there are a lot of lumps, a sifter or even a whisk can come in handy. A mortar and pestle is another item that can be used to remove lumps.

If you're following along with the recipe, take 2 cups of baking soda and mix one cup of citric acid into it now.

Step 2: Adding the Rest of the Dry Ingredients

There are a number of other dry ingredients that can be added to bath bombs, most of which are completely optional. Your only real limitation is your imagination. If it smells good and/or is good for your skin, there's a pretty good chance you can add it to your bath bombs to good effect.

I've seen all sorts of dry ingredients added to bath bombs. Here are just some of the many items people are adding to bath bombs these days:

Corn starch. Corn starch is one of the more common items added to bath bombs. It's added for one reason, and that's to make the bath bomb float. It's typically added in equal amounts to the amount of citric acid used, but that can vary based on the other dry ingredients added.

Dried flower petals. Flower petals that have been dried and crushed can be added to bath bombs to make them more interesting and to add fragrance to the bombs. They can be added and stirred in or sprinkled into the bottom of the mold, so that they're visible when the bath bombs are popped out.

Epsom salt. Epsom salt isn't actually a salt. It's a naturally-occurring mineral that's a mixture of sulfate and magnesium. The skin absorbs Epsom salt readily, and once inside the body it eases stress and helps you relax, while eliminating toxins and alleviating inflammation.

Herbs and spices. Dried herbs like oregano, mint, and cinnamon can be added to your bath bombs. Be careful not to add too much or your bath might end up smelling like a bowl of minestrone soup!

Salts. From Himalayan Sea Salt to Brazilian Salt to Coarse Pink Salt, there are all sorts of salts you can add to your bath bombs. They act as a gentle exfoliate when applied to the skin and add minerals to the tub water. Salts can be added during Step 2 and mixed into the bath bomb blend or they can be sprinkled into the bottom of the mold and used as a garnish that's visible when the bath bombs are popped out of the mold.

Sugars. While sugars are more commonly used in scrubs because they help exfoliate the skin, they can be added in small amounts to bath bombs to add a slightly-sweet smell to them. They can also be used as garnish for your bombs to add an interesting look to them.

Add the dry ingredients after you've thoroughly mixed the baking soda and citric acid together. Stir them in and you're ready to move on to the next step.

If you're following along, all we're going to add at this time is 1 cup of corn starch. Stir it in and make sure it's thoroughly mixed into the rest of the dry ingredients.

Remove any lumps that form before moving on to the next step.

Step 3: Combine the Wet Ingredients

There are three common types of wet ingredients that are added to bath bombs:

- **Butters.**
- **Dyes and other colorants.**
- **Essential Oils.**
- **Oils.**

We'll take a closer look at each of these ingredients individually in the coming sections, but for now just know they need to be combined before they're added to the bath bomb mixture.

Some of the butters and oils that are added to bath bombs are solids at cooler temperatures. Gently melt them over low heat and then add the rest of the wet ingredients and stir them in. Be careful not to heat the ingredients up too much or you can damage the oils. If all of the wet ingredients you're using are already in liquid form, you can add them to a jar, cap it and shake the jar to mix them together.

Don't worry too much about separation. The oils won't completely blend together and will start to separate as soon as they're mixed. Mix them up right before you add them to your bath bomb blend and you'll be good to go.

Those of you who are familiar with the bath bomb making process may have noticed one omission from the wet ingredients. I didn't include water or witch hazel in this step because I prefer to add this ingredient in a separate step in order to ensure my bath bomb blend is the right consistency.

If you're following along with this recipe, the only wet ingredients you're going to use are 2 tablespoons of olive oil and 5 drops of lavender essential oil. Combine them now.

Let's take a moment to explore the various oils, butters and essential oils that can be used to create bath bombs.

Carrier Oils

Carrier oils are added to bath bombs to help disperse the ingredients in the bath bomb throughout the entire water column in the tub. They also help carry essential oils beneath the surface of the skin, hence the name. Without carrier oils, all the oils in the bath bomb would float to the surface of the water and you'd get out of the tub feeling like you just jumped into an oil slick.

While they aren't anywhere near as powerful as essential oils, carrier oils carry with them (no pun intended) a number of benefits. The following carrier oils can all be used to make bath bombs:

Apricot kernel oil. This oil is derived from apricot pits and has a light, nutty fragrance that smells nothing like apricots. It's a lightweight oil that absorbs readily into the skin, moisturizing it and leaving it feeling soft and supple. Apricot kernel oil is ideal for dry, irritated skin or skin that's been ravaged by age or weather.

Avocado oil. Dry, aging skin appreciates the moisturizing and soothing properties of avocado oil. It's a heavy oil that penetrates deep beneath the skin to carry the vitamins and minerals it's rich with to the areas that need them most. Avocado oil has the light fragrance of avocadoes and must be used in small amounts when added to bath bombs because it's heavy and tends to leave a greasy sheen behind on the skin.

Castor oil. Thick and rich with nutrients and fatty acids, castor oil acts as a humectant that draws moisture into the skin. It has a light fragrance that smells slightly oily and is unlike the fragrance of any of the other oils.

Coconut oil. Coconut oil is solid at cooler temperatures, but once temperatures rise above 76° F, it will melt and become a liquid. It's important to keep this in mind when using coconut oil in bath bombs because using too much coconut oil can result in a bath bomb that melts as temperatures rise above its melting point. Coconut oil is a good choice for most skin types and is one of the more common oils used in bath bombs.

Jojoba oil. Jojoba oil isn't an oil at all. It's actually a liquid wax that's referred to as an oil in terms of the way it's used in personal care products. It helps moisturize the skin and has anti-inflammatory properties, as long as you don't mind feeling like you applied a fresh coat of Turtle Wax to your skin.

Grapeseed oil. This light oil is packed full of antioxidants and linoleic and oleic acids. It absorbs readily into the skin and is one of the few oils that leaves no residue on the skin after application. It's also odorless, which makes it a great option for lightly-scented bath bombs where other oils might overpower the fragrance of the essential oils you're using.

Olive oil. This is one oil you probably already have in the kitchen, since it's a common ingredient in a number of Western recipes. Olive oil gets the job done as a carrier oil, but there are usually other oils that will work better.

Sweet almond oil. This is a light oil that doesn't leave a residue behind and is readily absorbed into the skin. It has a light, nutty fragrance that's pleasant and won't overpower other fragrances. Sweet almond oil is one of my go-to oils for making bath bombs.

When adding carrier oils to bath bomb blends, it's important you make sure you don't add too much oil. If the mixture feels oily and greasy and is impossible to mold, you've added too much carrier oil. When this happens, you may be able to add more baking soda and citric acid to get it to the right consistency, but it's often easier to start over and try again.

Butters

Butters are an optional ingredient that can be used to firm up bath bombs and make them easier to mold. They also add a moisturizing effect to the bath bomb and may carry with them a handful of other benefits. If you're finding your bath bombs are crumbling like they're made of sand when you pull them out of the mold, adding a small amount of butter may help keep them stuck together.

There are a ton of specialty butters out there that you can spend a small fortune on. I've tried a number of them and they work fairly well, but I find I always end up coming back to just a small handful of less-expensive butters.

Here are the butters I use:

Aloe vera butter. Aloe vera butter isn't a true butter made from the aloe vera plant. It's made by mixing aloe vera oils with butters from other plants. The end result is a butter that's infused with the healing and regenerative properties of aloe vera.

Cocoa butter. This hard butter is made up of stable fats and is one of the top butters used in skin care products. It keeps the skin feeling soft, has moisturizing properties and is readily absorbed into the skin. It's created by pulling fatty acids out of cocoa beans and the butter smells like chocolate. What more could you ask for in an oil?

Mango butter. Mango butter is derived from the seeds of mangoes and is similar to cocoa butter in consistency. It has emollient and regenerative properties and is great for moisturizing and protecting the skin. It has a sweet fragrance, but sadly doesn't smell like the mangoes it's taken from.

Shea butter. This butter is softer than coconut butter and melts on contact with the skin. It works well for most skin types, but is especially beneficial to dry, damaged skin.

Essential Oils

Essential oils are volatile oils found in plants that give them their characteristic fragrance. They generally smell like the concentrated essence of the plant they're derived from. The main reason essential oils are added to bath bombs is to add fragrance to them, and they do this job well, filling the room with the amazing scents of great-smelling plants like roses, eucalyptus trees and your favorite herbs. Additionally, they carry with them a number of therapeutic benefits and are antimicrobial by nature.

Be aware that essential oils are extremely powerful compounds that can impact your body both positively and negatively depending on how they're used and the amount they're used in. When it comes to essential oils, less is more. That little bottle you just bought may not look like much, but it could contain the oil from as many as several thousand plants. While 10 to 20 drops of essential oil may not seem like much, it's more than enough to make your bath bomb smell great while providing a number of therapeutic benefits.

It's important you make sure any essential oils you decide to use in your bath bombs are safe to be applied to your skin. Some essential oils are known as "hot" oils, and they can cause burns similar to chemical burns in sensitive individuals. It's important to test any new oils you plan on using prior to using them in a bath bomb. Dilute a few drops of essential oil in a tablespoon of carrier oil and apply it to a small, inconspicuous area of your skin. Wait 24 hours and watch for irritation. If irritation occurs, don't use that oil in a bath bomb. Look at it this way. When you know you're allergic to certain foods, you don't eat them. If your body tells you it's allergic to certain essential oils, don't use them.

There are a number of essential oils that are considered safe for most people to use. Citrus oils, a number of wood oils, floral oils like lavender and rose oil and campherous oils are all used to good effect by a number of people. Check with your physician prior to adding a new essential oil to your bath bombs because there may be contraindications you aren't aware of.

Dyes

There are only a handful of dyes that can be used to make bath bombs. Unless you want to get out of the tub looking like Hellboy or a human Smurf, you should only use dyes that are skin-safe and won't change the color of your skin. Another concern is the tub, as some dyes will permanently dye your tub and anything else they come in contact with.

The best dyes to use for bath bombs are natural dyes that have been colorized with minerals and other compounds. Synthetic dyes are available, but I've always been a little leery about using them on my skin. I've heard of people using food coloring, but again, I worry about it coming in contact with my skin. I like to keep my bath bombs as natural as possible.

Step 4: Combine the Wet and the Dry Ingredients

You've got your wet and your dry ingredients mixed separately. Now what? Well, it's time to combine them, of course. Don't dump all of the wet ingredients into the dry ingredients at once. You'll end up setting off a reaction similar to those grade school volcanoes the cool kids brought to the science fair in 3rd grade.

Instead of dumping the wet ingredients in, you've got to add them slowly and whisk or stir them in. You'll know if you're adding them too fast because the baking soda and citric acid will start to bubble. If this happens, stir the bubbling portion of the blend into the rest of the blend and it should stop bubbling. Or it'll explode into a ball of scalding hot liquid, but that doesn't happen very often.

I was totally kidding about last part. Just checking to see if you're still paying attention.

Add the wet ingredients to the dry ingredients now and stir them in. Once they're combined and you've removed all the lumps, move on to the next step.

Step 5: Achieving the Right Consistency

In order to mold your bath bombs and to get them to hold their shape, the bath bomb blend has to be the proper consistency. It can't be too dry or it'll fall apart as soon as it comes out of the mold. On the other hand, it can't be too wet or it won't be moldable and you'll have trouble getting it to properly dry. There's nothing more frustrating than pulling a bath bomb out of a mold and having it crumble like it's made of sand the first time you bump it.

I've heard the consistency you're trying to achieve compared to wet sand, and that's a fairly accurate description. If you can grab a handful of the blend and squeeze it and it holds its shape when you release your grip, you're on the right track.

If you're lucky, you'll achieve this consistency after Step 4 is complete, but don't get your hopes up because that rarely happens. What usually ends up happening is the blend is too dry and you have to add liquid. There are two common liquids that can be added in this step. You can add water, witch hazel or a blend of water and witch hazel. I prefer witch hazel because it bubbles less when I accidentally spray too much.

You have to be really careful when adding liquid to your bath bomb blend in this step because it's easy to add too much. The best method I've found is to fill a spray bottle, set it to mist and spray several sprays onto the blend. I then stir it in and check the consistency. If it's still too dry, I'll add another spray or two and stir it in again. I continue doing this until the proper consistency is achieved.

Time for you to give it a try. Once you reach the right consistency, immediately move on to Step 6. Don't wait too long and give the blend time to dry.

Step 6: Molding

You've done the hard part. Now comes the fun part—pressing the bath bombs into the molds. The key to creating a working bath bomb is to get it packed into the mold as tightly as you can. Even if you do all of the previous steps correctly, messing this step up with a loose pack job will result in a bath bomb that falls apart in the tub, if it makes it there at all.

There are literally a ton of different items you can use as bath bombs molds. The easiest molds to pack tightly are those that come in two pieces. There are molds that are specially-made just for creating bath bombs that are extremely easy to use. All you have to do is fill both sides of the mold and then push the two halves together to create a tightly-packed bath bomb.

Other molds are open on one side. You fill these molds until they're over flowing and then flip them over and press them against a hard surface. There are also scoopers available that look like a pair scissors with half of a bath bomb mold on each end. This type of mold gives you more leverage to pack the bath bomb tightly. In a pinch, you can even use plastic Easter eggs as molds. Fill both halves and press them together until you're able to snap them shut.

The problem with molds that are made for bath bombs is there really aren't that many different varieties on the market. If you want to make anything other than stars, hearts or round balls, you're probably going to need to look elsewhere to find your molds. The good thing is there are a lot of options. You can use silicon molds, candy molds and any other plastic molds that are made from plastic. I've even seen people cut plastic Christmas ornaments in half and use them as molds.

Press your bath bombs into the molds and let them sit for a couple minutes before gently popping them out of the mold. Getting them in is easy. Removing them is the hard part and requires a little finesse. If you're using molds that have a lot of little details, you need to leave the bath bombs in the mold until they're completely dry or they'll break apart. Be careful when you're popping them out of the molds because they're fairly easy to dent and may crack or break apart if jostled too hard.

Step 7: Let the Bath Bombs Dry

This step's an easy one because you don't have to do anything. Leave the bath bombs sitting in a safe place in your home and give them time to dry. 8 to 12 hours is usually sufficient, but larger bath bombs may need more drying time.

And stop touching them. I know they look cool and you want to admire your handiwork, but they're best left alone in this step. If you've got young kids, put them up somewhere out of reach. Bath bombs look like they're fun to play with and kids love to play with them and roll them around.

Step 8: Storage

Bath bombs need to be kept in an airtight container. When I'm making bath bombs for home use, they go straight into a Tupperware container that can be sealed to protect them from the elements. If I don't have Tupperware available, I'll store them in sealable freezer bags.

I take a little more care when it comes to storing bath bombs I plan on selling or loaning to people. Mason jars work well when gifting multiple bath bombs. They can be gently stacked in the jar, and the jar can be adorned with a bow and a nice label to create an inexpensive gift that looks like it cost a pretty penny. They can also be individually-wrapped in cellophane and tied shut with ribbon.

Bath bombs should be used within 6 months of the day they're made in order to make sure the oils used in the bath bomb don't go rancid, but that usually isn't a concern in my house. I'm sure you'll use yours long before the 6 month mark. They're rather addicting.

Step 9: Using a Bath Bomb

Bath bombs are easy to use. Fill your tub up with warm water. Toss the bath bomb into the tub and it'll start bubbling. Well, it will if you made it properly. You can sit in the tub with the bath bomb as it bubbles and let the tiny bubbles gently caress your body or you can wait until the bath bomb is done fizzing to get in. As the bath bomb fizzes away to nothing, the oils and butters in the bomb will disperse into the tub and the fragrance of the essential oils you added will fill the room.

If you use a large bath bomb and it's still bubbling when you're ready to get out of the tub, you can take it out and use it again the next time you bathe. It'll look horrible, but should still work if you toss it back into the tub.

Do Not Use: Sodium Lauryl Sulfate (SLS)

Read enough literature on bath bombs and other homemade bath products and you'll eventually come across recipes that call for sodium lauryl sulfate (SLS). It's a chemical foaming agent that's used in commercial soaps, shampoos and other products we expect to foam. It's more a marketing ploy than anything, as the lather you see when you use these products doesn't do anything other than please the consumer.

Some people add it to their bath bomb recipes to help their bath bombs foam up, but it isn't really necessary. There's evidence that SLS can cause skin irritation and other issues when applied directly to the skin, so I'm not a big fan of soaking in a bathtub full of it. And to be completely honest, I tried it when I first starting making bath bombs and it really doesn't make that much of a difference...Definitely not enough for me to be willing to bathe in a tub full of it.

Skip the SLS and your body and skin will be all the better for it.

Practice Makes Perfect: The Basic Bath Bomb Recipe

This first recipe is about as basic as a bath bomb can get. No frills, no thrills and no fragrances so good they'll give you chills. All it really does is bubble and maybe moisturize your skin a bit. I'd recommend starting things off by working on creating this recipe until you've got it dialed in. If you followed along in the previous chapter, you're already a step ahead. If not, now's a good time to practice the basics. That way you don't end up wasting a bunch of the more expensive ingredients like the essential oils and butters.

As far as using these bath bombs goes, I'd say toss them in a large bowl of water or into a sink filled with warm water and make sure they fizz, but other than that, you aren't going to get much use out of them. If you want to make functional bath bombs, try blending 5 to 10 drops of lavender essential oil into the carrier oil.

Basic Bath Bomb Recipe

1 cup baking soda
½ cup citric acid
½ cup corn starch
2 tablespoons Epsom salt
1 teaspoon carrier oil
Water or witch hazel

Directions:

1. Combine the baking soda and the citric acid.
2. Add the corn starch and Epsom salt and mix them into the bath bomb blend.
3. There's only one wet ingredient, so you can skip to step 4.
4. Add the carrier oil to the bowl with the dry ingredients and stir it in. Use one of the lighter oils like coconut oil or even canola oil when starting out. Get rid of any lumps that form.
5. Check the consistency of the bath bomb blend. If it's too dry, mist water or witch hazel onto it and stir it in until it's the right consistency.
6. Press the bath bomb mixture into the molds.
7. Remove the bath bombs from the molds and let them dry.

Oatmeal Bombs

Growing up, I was always told not to play with my food, so I've always felt a little strange hopping into a tub that's full of ground oatmeal. My worries are soon forgotten, as the ground oatmeal dissolves in the tub water to create a soothing, milky bath that's great for all sorts of skin conditions, from dry skin to eczema to helping ease the pain associated with sunburns.

Be careful when climbing in and out of a tub with oatmeal in the water. The combination of oatmeal and the oils in the bathtub can create a slippery surface and you don't want to have to take a trip to the hospital (even though that is a great opportunity to show off your silky smooth skin).

This recipe leaves the choice of which essential oils to use up to you. If you're having trouble choosing which oils to use, 10 to 15 drops of lavender oil or rose geranium oil will get the job done nicely.

Oatmeal Bombs Recipe

1 cup baking soda
½ cup citric acid
½ cup oats
2 tablespoons Epsom salt
1 tablespoon Shea butter
Water or witch hazel
10 to 15 drops of your favorite essential oil blend

Directions:

1. Combine the baking soda and the citric acid.
2. Grind the oats in a spice grinder. Add the oats and Epsom salt to the baking soda and citric acid and mix them into the bath bomb blend.
3. Melt the Shea butter. Whisk the Shea butter and the essential oils together.
4. Add the essential oil and butter blend to the bowl with the dry ingredients and stir it in. Get rid of any lumps that form.
5. Check the consistency of the bath bomb blend. If it's too dry, mist water or witch hazel onto it and stir it in until it's the right consistency.
6. Press the bath bomb blend into the molds.
7. Remove the bath bombs from the molds and let them dry.
8. Store them in an airtight container until you're ready to use them.

Glitter Bombs

Glitter bombs are for those out there who want to get out of the tub sparkling with glitter and spend the rest of their day feeling like a beautiful princess. I don't recommend you use one of these before work unless you're a Disney princess or something along those lines. My teenage daughter loves using one of these bath bombs right before she has a school dance.

This bath bomb doesn't have any fragrances added. You can add your favorite oils or oil blends. I prefer floral oils with glitter bombs, with jasmine, rose otto and geranium oil being at the top of the list.

Glitter Bombs Recipe

1 cup baking soda
½ cup citric acid
¼ cup corn starch
2 tablespoons Epsom salt
1 tablespoon extra-virgin coconut oil
10 to 15 drops of your favorite essential oils
Shredded glitter
Water or witch hazel

Directions:

1. Combine the baking soda and the citric acid.
2. Add the corn starch and Epsom salt to the baking soda and citric acid and mix them into the bath

bomb blend. Add as much glitter as you'd like and stir it in.
3. Melt the coconut oil. Whisk the coconut oil and the essential oils together.
4. Add the oil blend to the bowl with the dry ingredients and stir it in. Get rid of any lumps that form.
5. Check the consistency of the bath bomb blend. If it's too dry, mist water or witch hazel onto it and stir it in until it's the right consistency.
6. Press the bath bomb blend into the molds.
7. Remove the bath bombs from the molds and let them dry.
8. Store them in an airtight container until you're ready to use them.

Rainbow Sherbet Bath Bombs

These bath bombs can either be molded into normal bath bomb molds or you can pack the bath bomb blend into a bowl and use a melon baller to remove little scoops that will look like scoops of rainbow sherbet ice cream.

As far as coloring goes, I usually use food coloring to get the vibrant green, orange and red colors needed to make them look like rainbow sherbet. This is one of the few times I make an exception to the "no chemicals" rule. You can use clays and other natural colorings if you'd like.

Rainbow Sherbet Bath Bombs Recipe

1 cup baking soda
½ cup citric acid
¼ cup corn starch
2 tablespoons Epsom salt
2 tablespoons extra-virgin coconut oil
5 drops lavender essential oil
5 drops lime essential oil
5 drops orange essential oil
Red, green and orange food dye (or natural colorings)
Water or witch hazel

Directions:

1. Combine the baking soda and the citric acid.
2. Add the corn starch and Epsom salt to the baking soda and citric acid and mix them into the bath bomb blend.

3. Melt the coconut oil. Whisk the coconut oil and the essential oils together.
4. Add the essential oil and coconut oil blend to the bowl with the dry ingredients and stir it in. Get rid of any lumps that form.
5. Check the consistency of the bath bomb blend. If it's too dry, mist water or witch hazel onto it and stir it in until it's the right consistency.
6. Divide the bath bomb blend into three equal portions. Color one of the portions pink, one green and one orange.
7. Press the bath bomb blend into the molds, adding a little bit of each color. Remove the bath bombs from the molds. Alternatively, press the bath bomb blend into a shallow bowl in rows of color and use a melon baller to remove scoops that look like little ice cream scoops.
8. Let the bath bombs dry overnight.
9. Store them in an airtight container until you're ready to use them.

Lovely Lavender

The next bath bomb we're going to make adds two ingredients. This recipe requires lavender essential oil and dried lavender flowers. I chose lavender essential oil because it's one of the safest essential oils around, and most people can tolerate it.

If you've never smelled lavender flowers or lavender essential oil, it can be a bit off-putting at first. It's going to be unlike anything you've ever smelled, and the fragrance might take some getting used to. Try adding a couple drops to the palms of your hands and holding them up to your nose while you breathe deeply. The fragrance of lavender is calming and soothing, and most people learn to love it.

Lavender essential oil has healing properties and is a great oil for most skin types, but is especially beneficial to dry or damaged skin. I toss a lavender bomb in the tub and ease myself in when I have a sunburn. It usually alleviates much of the pain and I rarely peel.

If you want to dye these bath bombs purple to match the color of lavender flowers, try using a purple mineral mica dye.

Lovely Lavender Recipe

1 cup baking soda
½ cup citric acid
½ cup corn starch
2 tablespoons Epsom salt
2 tablespoons sweet almond oil
10 to 15 drops lavender essential oil

Dried lavender
Water or witch hazel

Directions:

1. Combine the baking soda and the citric acid.
2. Add the corn starch and Epsom salt and mix them into the bath bomb blend.
3. Combine the sweet almond oil and the lavender essential oil and whisk them together.
4. Add the oil blend to the bowl with the dry ingredients and stir it in. Get rid of any lumps that form.
5. Check the consistency of the bath bomb blend. If it's too dry, mist water or witch hazel onto it and stir it in until it's the right consistency.
6. Crumble the lavender flowers. Add a small amount of the flowers to the bottom of each mold. Press the bath bomb mixture into the molds.
7. Remove the bath bombs from the molds and let them dry.
8. Store them in an airtight container until you're ready to use them.

Tea Tree Oil Bath Bomb

Tea tree oil used to be something nobody other than aromatherapists were familiar with, but it's been pulled into the mainstream lately and there have been a number of hair and skin care products containing it hitting the market of late. If you've already purchased one of these products, you know what to expect as far as fragrance goes. If not, be prepared to be surprised. The fragrance is campherous and slightly minty, and it punches you right in the sinus cavity. Like lavender, it isn't a fragrance most people instantly love and can take some getting used to.

Where tea tree oil really comes into its own is in the skin care department. It's antibacterial, antiviral and antifungal by nature and can be used to fight off infections, rashes and has seen use as a home remedy for respiratory conditions. Try adding 5 to 10 drops of lavender oil to this recipe to up the skin care properties even more.

Spirulina powder can be added to these bath bombs to dye them an interesting green color.

Tea Tree Oil Bath Bomb Recipe

1 cup baking soda
½ cup citric acid
½ cup corn starch
2 tablespoons Epsom salt
2 tablespoons sweet almond oil
10 to 15 drops tea tree essential oil
Water or witch hazel

Directions:

1. Combine the baking soda and the citric acid.
2. Add the corn starch and Epsom salt and mix them into the bath bomb blend.
3. Combine the sweet almond oil and the tea tree essential oil and whisk them together.
4. Add the oil blend to the bowl with the dry ingredients and stir it in. Get rid of any lumps that form.
5. Check the consistency of the bath bomb blend. If it's too dry, mist water or witch hazel onto it and stir it in until it's the right consistency.
6. Press the bath bomb mixture into the molds.
7. Remove the bath bombs from the molds and give them time to dry. Depending on how damp the mixture is, this can take up to 24 hours.
8. Store them in an airtight container until you're ready to use them.

Candy Cane Bath Bombs

If you've ever eaten a candy cane or one of those little red and white peppermints, then you know what peppermint essential oil smells like. This essential oil is a powerful oil that's strongly antimicrobial and benefits the skin in a number of ways. It brightens dull and fading skin while exfoliating and toning it and can be used to control the excretion of oils by the skins pores.

Peppermint oil doesn't just benefit the skin. The fragrance of peppermint oil will leave you feeling energized and refreshed. If you've got a cold or some other minor respiratory issue, taking deep breaths while you're in the bath may help clear up congestion and ease coughing.

Be aware peppermint oil is a strong oil and isn't tolerated by everyone. All essential oils should be tested on a small area of the skin prior to use, but this is especially-critical with peppermint oil.

Candy Cane Bath Bomb Recipe

1 cup baking soda
½ cup citric acid
½ cup corn starch
2 tablespoons Epsom salt
1 tablespoon sweet almond oil
15 drops peppermint essential oil
Mint sprigs
Water or witch hazel
OPTIONAL: Natural pink clay, for pink coloring

Directions:

1. Combine the baking soda and the citric acid.
2. Add the corn starch and Epsom salt and mix them into the bath bomb blend. Add a small amount of pink clay at this time and stir it in, if you plan on coloring the bath bombs.
3. Whisk the sweet almond oil and peppermint essential oil together.
4. Add the oil and butter blend to the bowl with the dry ingredients and stir it in. Get rid of any lumps that form.
5. Check the consistency of the bath bomb blend. If it's too dry, mist water or witch hazel onto it and stir it in until it's the right consistency.
6. Add a mint sprig to the bottom of each bath bomb mold and press the bath bomb blend into the molds.
7. Remove the bath bombs from the molds and let them dry.
8. Store them in an airtight container until you're ready to use them.

Pink Grapefruit Bath Bombs

The pink grapefruit bath bomb is one of my personal favorites. It's a simple bath bomb to make, and for some reason, it makes me feel like I'm sitting in a tub full of Squirt soda…minus the sugar and uncomfortable stickiness, of course.

Pink grapefruit essential oil is astringent and helps tighten up the skin. It's got a refreshing fragrance that's uplifting and will leave your mind, body and skin feeling rejuvenated.

Pink Grapefruit Bath Bomb Recipe

1 cup baking soda
½ cup citric acid
½ cup corn starch
2 tablespoons Epsom salt
1 tablespoon extra-virgin coconut oil
10 drops pink grapefruit essential oil
Water or witch hazel
OPTIONAL: Natural pink clay, for pink coloring

Directions:

1. Combine the baking soda and the citric acid.
2. Add the corn starch and Epsom salt and mix them into the bath bomb blend. Add a small amount of pink clay at this time and stir it in, if you plan on coloring the bath bombs.

3. Melt the coconut oil. Whisk the coconut oil and pink grapefruit essential oil together.
4. Add the oil blend to the bowl with the dry ingredients and stir it in. Get rid of any lumps that form.
5. Check the consistency of the bath bomb blend. If it's too dry, mist water or witch hazel onto it and stir it in until it's the right consistency.
6. Press the bath bombs into the molds.
7. Remove the bath bombs from the molds and let them dry.
8. Store them in an airtight container until you're ready to use them.

Pear Bath Bombs

There are those who claim to have gotten their hands on pear essential oil, but if it does exist, I've never seen it. Other sources say it doesn't exist. I'm assuming that if it did, it would be extremely expensive due to its rarity.

In order to get the pear fragrance in this bath bomb, I turned to organic pear fragrance oil, which was the next best thing. It definitely doesn't feature the therapeutic benefits that essential oils have, but it does have a great pear fragrance that isn't overpowering like some synthetic fragrances.

Pear Bath Bombs Recipe

1 cup baking soda
½ cup citric acid
½ cup corn starch
2 tablespoons Epsom salt
1 tablespoon sweet almond oil
10 to 15 drops organic pear fragrance oil
Water or witch hazel
OPTIONAL: Natural green coloring

Directions:

1. Combine the baking soda and the citric acid.
2. Add the corn starch and Epsom salt and mix them into the bath bomb blend. Add a small amount of natural green coloring at this time and stir it in, if you plan on coloring the bath bombs.

3. Whisk the sweet almond oil and pear fragrance oil together.
4. Add the oil blend to the bowl with the dry ingredients and stir it in. Get rid of any lumps that form.
5. Check the consistency of the bath bomb blend. If it's too dry, mist water or witch hazel onto it and stir it in until it's the right consistency.
6. Remove the bath bombs from the molds and let them dry.
7. Store them in an airtight container until you're ready to use them.

Rose Petal Surprise

Rose otto oil is an expensive essential oil because it takes thousands of roses to produce just a small amount. Just a couple ounces of this oil can run you upwards of $50. If you can afford it, rose otto oil is worth the investment because it provides a luxurious, relaxing bath time experience when it's added to bath bombs. You're only going to be using 10 to 15 drops of the oil each time you make the recipe, so a little vial will last a long time.

If you can't afford rose otto oil, or you just don't want to pay the price, you can substitute rose geranium oil in this recipe. It's a similar oil that's a little bit cheaper. It doesn't quite provide the same experience, but gets the job done.

Rose Petal Surprise Recipe

1 cup baking soda
½ cup citric acid
¼ cup corn starch
2 tablespoons Epsom salt
1 tablespoon Shea butter
5 drops lavender essential oil
10 drops rose otto essential oil
Water or witch hazel
Dried rose petals

Directions:

1. Combine the baking soda and the citric acid.

2. Add the corn starch and Epsom salt to the baking soda and citric acid and mix them into the bath bomb blend.
3. Melt the Shea butter. Whisk the Shea butter and the essential oils together.
4. Add the essential oil and butter blend to the bowl with the dry ingredients and stir it in. Get rid of any lumps that form.
5. Check the consistency of the bath bomb blend. If it's too dry, mist water or witch hazel onto it and stir it in until it's the right consistency.
6. Add a few rose petals to the bottom of the bath bomb mold.
7. Press the bath bomb blend into the molds. Once you've filled half the mold, make a depression in the bath bomb and fill it with rose petals. Finish filling the mold with the bath bomb blend. The idea is to make a bath bomb that releases the rose petals once it's been in the tub for a while.
8. Remove the bath bombs from the molds and let them dry.
9. Store them in an airtight container until you're ready to use them.

Taste of the Tropics Bath Bomb

Here's a bath bomb that's simple to make, yet smells like you used a blend of essential oils to create a floral fragrance that's exotic and evokes thoughts of the tropics. The secret is frangipani essential oil, which comes from the flowers and other parts of the plumeria tree. It's a floral oil with hints of roses, pineapple, banana and all sorts of other good fragrances. The fragrance manages to be both relaxing and revitalizing at the same time.

The benefits of frangipani oil don't stop at the great smell. It's said to have age-defying effects and is thought to revitalize the skin and hair. It has anti-inflammatory properties that will help eliminate rashes and inflammation, and the moisturizing properties help make the skin smoother and softer.

Taste of the Tropics Recipe

1 cup baking soda
½ cup citric acid
¼ cup corn starch
2 tablespoons Epsom salt
1 tablespoon extra-virgin coconut oil
15 drops frangipani essential oil
Water or witch hazel

Directions:

1. Combine the baking soda and the citric acid.

2. Add the corn starch and Epsom salt to the baking soda and citric acid and mix them into the bath bomb blend.
3. Melt the coconut oil. Whisk the coconut oil and the frangipani essential oil together.
4. Add the oil blend to the bowl with the dry ingredients and stir it in. Get rid of any lumps that form.
5. Check the consistency of the bath bomb blend. If it's too dry, mist water or witch hazel onto it and stir it in until it's the right consistency.
6. Press the bath bomb blend into the molds.
7. Remove the bath bombs from the molds and let them dry.
8. Store them in an airtight container until you're ready to use them.

Summer Breeze

I'll be the first to admit this bath bomb isn't going to be loved by everyone. Sweetgrass essential oil has a unique fragrance that's light and airy with hints of fresh-cut grass. It's extremely relaxing, so a short soak is all you need. Sweetgrass oil can be a bit tough to find locally, but it can usually be sourced online.

These bath bombs can be dyed green using natural clays.

Summer Breeze Bath Bomb Recipe

1 cup baking soda
½ cup citric acid
½ cup corn starch
2 tablespoons Epsom salt
1 tablespoon sweet almond oil
5 drops sweetgrass essential oil
Water or witch hazel

Directions:

1. Combine the baking soda and the citric acid.
2. Add the corn starch and Epsom salt to the baking soda and citric acid and mix them into the bath bomb blend.
3. Whisk the sweet almond oil and the sweetgrass essential oil together.
4. Add the oil blend to the bowl with the dry ingredients and stir it in. Get rid of any lumps that form.

5. Check the consistency of the bath bomb blend. If it's too dry, mist water or witch hazel onto it and stir it in until it's the right consistency.
6. Press the bath bomb blend into the molds.
7. Remove the bath bombs from the molds and let them dry.
8. Store them in an airtight container until you're ready to use them.

Hot Chocolate Bomb

If you love chocolate milk, you're going to love this bath bomb because it makes you feel like you're a marshmallow floating smack dab in the middle of a tub full of hot cocoa. Just make sure you don't give in to temptation and drink some of the bath water. It won't taste anywhere near as good as it smells!

Hot Chocolate Bomb Recipe

1 cup baking soda
½ cup citric acid
¼ cup corn starch
2 tablespoons Epsom salt
2 tablespoons cacao powder
2 tablespoons cocoa butter
Water or witch hazel

Directions:

1. Combine the baking soda and the citric acid.
2. Add the corn starch and Epsom salt to the baking soda and citric acid and mix them into the bath bomb blend.
3. Melt the cocoa butter.
4. Add the melted butter to the bowl with the dry ingredients and stir it in. Get rid of any lumps that form.

5. Check the consistency of the bath bomb blend. If it's too dry, mist water or witch hazel onto it and stir it in until it's the right consistency.
6. Press the bath bomb blend into the molds. Layer the bath bomb blend and thin layers of cacoa powder to create a marbled effect.
7. Remove the bath bombs from the molds and let them dry.
8. Store them in an airtight container until you're ready to use them.

Skin Softening Bath Bomb

This bath bomb will work for most skin types, but it's especially beneficial to those who have dry, damaged skin or skin that's been ravaged by age or weather. It combines cocoa butter, Shea butter and coconut oil to create an oil and butter blend that will leave even the roughest skin feeling soft and supple.

The skin softening bath bomb doesn't call for any essential oils and features the slight fragrance of chocolate and coconut on its own. You can use it like this, or you can add your own blend of essential oils to the mix to make it smell great while adding additional therapeutic properties.

Skin Softening Bath Bomb Recipe

1 cup baking soda
½ cup citric acid
½ cup corn starch
2 tablespoons Epsom salt
1 tablespoon cocoa butter
1 tablespoon Shea butter
2 tablespoons extra-virgin coconut oil
Water or witch hazel
OPTIONAL: 10 to 15 drops of your favorite essential oil blend

Directions:

1. Combine the baking soda and the citric acid.

2. Add the corn starch and Epsom salt and mix them into the bath bomb blend.
3. Melt the cocoa butter, Shea butter and coconut oil. Whisk them together. If you're using essential oils, add them and stir them in.
4. Add the oil and butter blend to the bowl with the dry ingredients and stir it in. Get rid of any lumps that form.
5. Check the consistency of the bath bomb blend. If it's too dry, mist water or witch hazel onto it and stir it in until it's the right consistency.
6. Press the bath bomb blend into the molds.
7. Remove the bath bombs from the molds and let them dry.
8. Store them in an airtight container until you're ready to use them.

Skin Toning Bath Bomb

Lactic acid treatments are an expensive spa treatment used to tone and tighten aging skin. This bath bomb creates a similar effect to a lactic acid treatment at a fraction of the price. It uses powdered milk, which is a natural source of lactic acid. When applied to the skin, it tightens things up a bit and smooths out wrinkles. It also helps close up large pores.

This recipe adds eucalyptus and myrrh essential oils to further enhance the skin tightening and toning power. If you don't have these essential oils on hand, you can use lavender oil or pretty much any other essential oil or oil blend you have available. Citrus oils are another good choice for tightening and toning the skin.

Skin Toning Bath Bomb Recipe

1 cup baking soda
½ cup citric acid
¼ cup corn starch
¼ cup powdered milk
1 tablespoon Jojoba oil
10 drops myrrh essential oil
5 drops eucalyptus essential oil
Water or witch hazel

Directions:

1. Combine the baking soda and the citric acid.

2. Add the corn starch, powdered milk and Epsom salt and mix them into the bath bomb blend.
3. Melt the Jojoba oil. Combine the Jojoba oil and the essential oils and whisk them together.
4. Add the oil blend to the bowl with the dry ingredients and stir it in. Get rid of any lumps that form.
5. Check the consistency of the bath bomb blend. If it's too dry, mist water or witch hazel onto it and stir it in until it's the right consistency.
6. Press the bath bomb mixture into the molds.
7. Remove the bath bombs from the molds and let them dry.
8. Store them in an airtight container until you're ready to use them.

The Awakening

Sometimes it can be tough to get going, especially later on in the week when you've been burning the candle at both ends. The Awakening bath bomb is designed to be used in the morning before you head out for the day because it will leave you feeling awake and refreshed. It's also a great bath bomb to use when you're feeling down in the dumps.

The Awakening Recipe

1 cup baking soda
½ cup citric acid
¼ cup corn starch
2 tablespoons Epsom salt
1 tablespoon extra-virgin coconut oil
5 drops orange essential oil
5 drops lemongrass essential oil
Water or witch hazel

Directions:

1. Combine the baking soda and the citric acid.
2. Add the corn starch and Epsom salt to the baking soda and citric acid and mix them into the bath bomb blend.
3. Melt the coconut oil. Whisk the coconut oil and the essential oils together.
4. Add the oil blend to the bowl with the dry ingredients and stir it in. Get rid of any lumps that form.

5. Check the consistency of the bath bomb blend. If it's too dry, mist water or witch hazel onto it and stir it in until it's the right consistency.
6. Press the bath bomb blend into the molds.
7. Remove the bath bombs from the molds and let them dry.
8. Store them in an airtight container until you're ready to use them.

The Goodnight Bomb

This bath bomb is the polar opposite of The Awakening bath bomb. It's designed to help you relax and unwind after a long day, and should help you wind down up to the point where you're ready for bed.

Don't use this bomb in the mornings if you've got a long day ahead. You might find you're drowsy and groggy all day!

The Goodnight Bomb Recipe

1 cup baking soda
½ cup citric acid
¼ cup corn starch
2 tablespoons Epsom salt
1 tablespoon extra-virgin coconut oil
10 drops lavender essential oil
5 drops ylang ylang essential oil
Water or witch hazel

Directions:

1. Combine the baking soda and the citric acid.
2. Add the corn starch and Epsom salt to the baking soda and citric acid and mix them into the bath bomb blend.
3. Melt the coconut oil. Whisk the coconut oil and the essential oils together.

4. Add the oil blend to the bowl with the dry ingredients and stir it in. Get rid of any lumps that form.
5. Check the consistency of the bath bomb blend. If it's too dry, mist water or witch hazel onto it and stir it in until it's the right consistency.
6. Press the bath bomb blend into the molds.
7. Remove the bath bombs from the molds and let them dry.
8. Store them in an airtight container until you're ready to use them.

Printed in Great Britain
by Amazon